Exercise Equipment: Selecting the Best for Cardio Workouts

What You Need To Know Before Buying Exercise Equipment for Cardio Workouts

By: Barry Cromer

9781630225780

I0414101

TABLE OF CONTENTS

PUBLISHERS NOTES

Speedy Publishing LLC

40 E. Main St., #1156

Newark, DE 19711

www.speedypublishing.co

Cover Artwork: 24 Hr. Designs Ltd.

Editing: Speedy Publishing LLC

Book design: Speedy Publishing LLC

ISBN: 9781630225780

This is a reprint book.

DISCLAIMER

This publication is intended to provide helpful and informative material. It is not intended to diagnose, treat, cure, or prevent any health problem or condition, nor is intended to replace the advice of a physician. No action should be taken solely on the contents of this book. Always consult your physician or qualified health-care professional on any matters regarding your health and before adopting any suggestions in this book or drawing inferences from it.

The author and publisher specifically disclaim all responsibility for any liability, loss or risk, personal or otherwise, which is incurred as a consequence, directly or indirectly, from the use or application of any contents of this book.

Any and all product names referenced within this book are the trademarks of their respective owners. None of these owners have sponsored, authorized, endorsed, or approved this book.

Always read all information provided by the manufacturers' product labels before using their products. The author and publisher are not responsible for claims made by manufacturers.

DEDICATION

To my uncle Bobby - If it wasn't for you wanting to buy exercise equipment and asking for my help, I wouldn't have known so much about what's actually involved beforehand. Thanks!

CHAPTER 1- WHAT YOU SHOULD KNOW ABOUT CARDIO EXERCISE EQUIPMENT

There are many concepts and facts you should know about cardio exercise equipment.

Weight loss is an important topic in almost all online forums. Fitness gyms are enjoying huge growth in their memberships. Many consumer products are now offering simple solutions to help people control and lose excessive weight. Everyone simply is into effective weight loss. Experts recommend cardiovascular exercises. Not surprisingly, there are now many and different cardio exercise equipment sold across the market. Such machines vary by brand and by type.

Do you think you need cardio exercise equipment? If you have excessive weight and bulging body fats, you surely are certain about your need to invest in such machines. It is not just another fad, although some people treat it as one. You should decide to tediously and strictly use your cardio exercise equipment if you want to make use of it. Make your investment matter. Such machines are not cheap. That is why you surely would strive to use them to their maximum.

There are many concepts and facts you should know about cardio exercise equipment. Before you go to any retailer to find and buy the best possible cardio machine there is, you should pause for a while and make practical assessments of yourself and of the equipment you are eyeing. What should you know about such cardio exercise machines?

First, be reminded that your body is still the ultimate and best cardio exercise machine. Experts keep on reminding people that any cardio exercise would always be effective if there is enough motivation and determination to perform them. Any machine would not be useful and successful if you would not take the resolve to use it. And there is a need to use cardio exercise equipment correctly and appropriately if you intend to make the use out of it.

Such machines could add fun and excitement to weight training in general. You may opt not to invest in one because you could perform other cardio exercises without the aid of equipment. However, if you really want to increase your motivation and condition your body and mind to do exercises, you should buy and use appropriate cardio exercise equipment now.

What is the main purpose of all cardio exercise equipment? You may have a quick impression that such machines are designed and marketed to help people lose excessive weight. You are correct in one way. But do you understand how the equipment could do that? Cardio exercises facilitated by such machines tend to move every muscle in the body.

In the process, more oxygen is used up by the muscles during an exercise. The heart would be prompted to pump more blood. The heart rate rises in the process. In the same way, metabolism is accelerated and more stored calories in the body are consumed. Thus, cardio exercise equipment help make people get back to shape. If you are familiar about such machines, you would know which one would help you achieve your goals and make you maximize the effective cardiovascular exercise.

CHAPTER 2- ALTERNATIVE CARDIO EXERCISE EQUIPMENT

When you talk about cardio exercise equipment, there are just a few popular machines that immediately come into your mind. For sure they include the treadmill, the elliptical machines, the rowing machines, and the stationary bike. You should be reminded that there are still more cardio exercise machines available. It is just that the abovementioned ones are the most popular. They are also the most commonly found in gyms and fitness centers. If you do not enjoy using any of those, you may take a look at alternative or less popular cardio exercise equipment around.

Stair masters are actually more like treadmills. The only difference is that stair masters are used to facilitate climbing motion of your legs. Efficiency is easily achieved because the body weight is used to further push the steps down. Increasing the level of difficulty could pose greater challenge to bring about bigger cardio advantage.

Stair mills or step mills are usually described as 'escalators coming from hell'. They are used as if you are stepping up local stadium steps. However, such steps may seem never ending. Step mills are more recommended to beginners. Even at lower settings, the machines could make the heart beat much faster. Increasing the level of difficulty would make the escalator go much faster so beware.

Versa climbers are among the best and most challenging cardio exercise equipment around. In general, this machine is among the least popular among cardio machines in almost every gym. Do not be surprised if you find it unused and just collecting dust. However, it is a very good cardio tool. It facilitates a movement as if you are climbing vertically. You would be forced to go against the natural gravity. The use of the machine could easily and effectively increase your heart rate.

Tread climbers are among the newest cardio exercise machines in the market. Manufacturers claim that the equipment is the best cardio exercise. Needless to say, tread climbers are combining the wonders of a treadmill and climbing equipment. You could not run on this one. You could only walk. However, the calories burned are much greater. When using this, remember not to put most of your body weight to the handles. To be safe, hold the handles firmly on your first try.

The arc trainer is non-impact cardio exercise equipment. You would be asked to step on 2 platforms. Start swinging your legs back and then forth. There is an adjustable resistance so you could better use speed. Non-impact cardio machines are best recommended for people suffering from chronic joint problems.

Lastly, hand ergometers are cardio exercise equipment for the handicapped. The item is highly recommended for people with broken legs, surgically repaired knee, and sprained ankle. In general, hand ergometers are better in increasing heart rates than almost any other cardio exercise equipment. This is because the arms, which are targeted by the machine, are logically closer to the heart than the legs. The machine is not exclusive to people with leg disabilities, though.

CHAPTER 3- MORE ON CARDIO EXERCISE EQUIPMENT

When planning to engage in cardio exercises it's not enough that you know the equipment. What's more important is that you are aware of the physiological processes that occur during each routine.

The heart is like a person. The muscles have to be strengthened in order to perform physical tasks. Now since the heart is the organ responsible for pumping blood throughout the body's system then it should be exposed to various cardio trainings via different exercise equipment.

There are lots of machines and devices available in your local gym and sporting goods store. The treadmill has been around for quite some time. It offers a rotating belt that allows you to walk, jog, and run your way towards a healthy heart.

A modified version of the treadmill is the elliptical machine. You ride a platform and swing your legs back and forth to obtain the desired heart rate for proper conditioning. It has an additional benefit of not putting your joints under wear and tear situations.

Climbing a flight of stairs can trigger your heart to pump faster. This is mimicked by a machine called the stair climber. It can pose a more challenging routine as compared to the regular treadmill and elliptical machine.

You can ride your way towards a strong heart via stationary cycles. There are recumbent models that allow you as well to have a more relaxed posture thus preventing lower back straining. Rowing machines are also present in gyms which give you the chance to heighten your heart's capacity by simulating boat rowing.

You have been introduced to the various cardio machines that are involved in standard training sessions but do you know how such contraptions really affect the functioning of your heart? Routines performed on these machines boost the strength and conditioning of your heart by increasing your heart rate for a given period. Actually it's the large muscle groups at work that really tell your heart to do extra pumps. Each activity of these muscles demand increased oxygen supply and the only way to deliver this oxygen requirement is by delivering more blood to the muscles.

Now that you have a clearer physiological picture, let's go to the factors that may affect your choice of cardio equipment. You have to build a certain liking for the machine. You won't be productive if you're not enjoying the company of the contraption. At this point your efforts are useless and you don't get maximum benefits.

You have to determine if you have a certain condition that will only be exaggerated once you perform your routines on a machine. If you have joint problems in your lower extremity then the treadmill might not work to your advantage. You have an office work and you remain idle on your seat for the whole day then the stationary bike won't be compatible with your needs.

Another thing to look at when you deal with machines is the actual time that you spend on it. You have to allot a good five to ten minutes of warm-up time before going to your actual routine making sure that intensity levels are kept low. Afterwards you can proceed to the workout that may last from twenty to sixty minutes basically depending on your preference. You close the deal with another five to ten minutes of low intensity warm-down time. Machine usage should be scheduled three to five times weekly.

Barry Cromer

When planning to engage in cardio exercises it's not enough that you know the equipment. What's more important is that you are aware of the physiological processes that occur during each routine. A good assessment of what you need and should avoid is a plus.

CHAPTER 4- CAN A CARDIO EXERCISE EQUIPMENT ENHANCE YOUR METABOLISM

While it is true that the use of cardio exercise equipment will enhance metabolism and overall health, you must remember that too much cardio is bad for your health.

Coupled with healthy diet and lifestyle, cardio exercises like walking, cycling, running, or jogging can increase your heart health and enhance your body's metabolism. Cardio exercises can be done indoors or outdoors. If you're a busy person, you might prefer an indoor training (in a fitness gym or at home) than outdoor training. Here's a brief overview of the most popular types of cardio exercise equipment you can use or buy to improve your overall health:

1. Treadmills - This machine lets you walk, run, or jog in a smooth, very predictable terrain. Treadmills yield a wide variety of choices and can be programmed depending on your needs. If you're just starting out, you can walk at a slow pace on level surface. As you progress, you can increase either the pace or incline so you can burn more fats and keep your heart rate in your target zone.

Compare to running outdoors, a treadmill pulls the ground underneath your feet so running is made somewhat easier. The cushioning in treadmills helps minimize stress on your joints. If you will run on the treadmill, it is best to look for one that has speed up to 10 mph and a longer deck to accommodate a longer stride. If you will walk on the treadmill, it is recommended to look for one with a maximum speed of 5 mph and a deck that is of average length.

2. Elliptical Trainers - An elliptical trainer lets you do a workout as intense as running or cross-country skiing but without any of the impact. Elliptical trainers are not weight bearers, so it's gentle on the joints and provides a very fluid movement.

Elliptical trainers provide a variety of configurations. If you want to simulate walking or running up hills, it is best to try a machine that has an incline option. If you want to adjust the intensity of your workout, you may pedal faster, raise the incline, and increase the resistance or any combination of machine's features.

3. Stationary Bikes - This cardio exercise equipment is especially designed for cycling which is considered by many fitness experts as the safest cross-training activity. Stationary bikes are also not weight bearers and can really help increase your endurance. Stationary bikes come in two varieties: upright and recumbent. Upright bikes imitate a regular bike while recumbent bikes let you sit in a slightly reclining position.

If you want a more steadily paced fat-burning workout, you can keep the resistance of your bike fairly low and spin the pedals faster. If you consider yourself already in advanced phase and your stationary bike has preprogrammed features, you may try the hill-climbing or interval option to enhance calorie burn. You may also try to simulate climbing a hill by manually increasing the resistance for a few minutes and then decreasing it.

According to the book "Make Over Your Metabolism" by Robert Reames, you can "manage your weight, shape, and appetite by providing a time-efficient, fat-burning exercise plan, a super simple nutrition plan that will optimize your metabolism, and lifestyle strategies that will help correct red flags that interfere with a healthy metabolism." While it is true that the use of cardio exercise equipment in performing training to enhance metabolism and overall health, you must remember that too much cardio is bad for your health.

Thus, many fitness experts recommend that a 30-minute cardio exercise is enough to keep your metabolism healthy.

CHAPTER 5- CARDIO EXERCISE EQUIPMENT BASIC TYPES

There are many types of cardio equipment but they can be grouped into five main categories.

Buying cardio exercise equipment is a big investment, that's why it is important to take time to research to determine the right machine that will suit your fitness health. Here's an overview of the basic types of cardio exercise equipment:

1. Stationary bikes are designed for people who prefer sitting than standing while burning calories. If you prefer the comfort of cycling than walking, rowing, or jogging for cardiovascular fitness, toning or building of your thighs; stationary bikes is for you. The stationary bike is a great leg builder; it will help strengthen your quadriceps muscles, the gluteus muscles, and the hamstring muscles.

There are two types of stationary bikes: the upright bikes and recumbent bikes. Upright bikes simulate a regular bike; the only difference is that it will not let you go anywhere. Recumbent bikes, on the other hand, have bucket seats so you pedal out in front of you. If you are new to exercise or prefer more back support because of a lower-back pain, you may find a recumbent bike more comfortable to use than an upright bike.

2. Stair climber is an excellent workout machine for your calves, thighs, hips, buttocks, and lowers back. If you prefer more than just walking and jogging, a stair climber is for you. However, it is important to consult your doctor first if you have previous or preexisting knee problem as it may exacerbate your injury. Stair climbers come in two types: with dependent steppers and with independent steppers. If you are a beginner, it is advised to use the

dependent stepper type as it is easier to use than the independent stepper type. The intensity of workout can be adjusted manually or through computer controls.

3. Rowing machines help strengthen your arms, legs, shoulders, and back with very low impact. However, it is not advised to people with back problem and even those with healthy backs are cautioned as it can strain muscles from rowing. Rowing machines have different types of resistance. Standard rowing machines use air resistance, other models use a water flywheel which is more closer to real rowing, and still other models use pistons or cylinders. Among of the best stair climbers are the ones with comfortable, adjustable seat and footpads; a bar with easy and comfortable grip; and with low noise.

4. Elliptical trainers are like the treadmill, they are designed to mimic the human gait during locomotion. However, compare to treadmill, this machine doesn't require your feet to leave the pedals which make it feel like you are running on a cloud. Elliptical trainers are recommended to people who suffer from lower-limb injuries or arthritis. The drive system of an elliptical machine is the mechanism by which it applies resistance during exercise. There are two basic types: front drive and rear drive.

5. Treadmill is probably the top seller among types of cardio exercise equipment. This machine offer an ideal way to increase your cardiovascular capacity, burn calories, and strengthen your lower body by allowing you to run and walk. Unlike walking or running outdoors, exercises with treadmills minimize stress on your joints. The shock is absorbed by the treadmill's cushioned deck. If you are overweight or have joint problems, fitness experts advise to look for a deck with more cushioning, preferably 18 inches wide or more.

CHAPTER 6- CARDIO EXERCISE EQUIPMENT FOR THE ELDERLY

Exercise is extremely important for the elderly as it prevents the onset or worsening of certain debilitating diseases like osteoporosis and heart disease.

Exercise is not just for the young. Everybody benefits from regular exercise and activity, even if you are more than 65 years old. Regular cardiovascular exercises would help improve your mood, lower risks of injury and protects your body from chronic diseases like heart disease and high blood pressure. However, your choice of cardio exercise equipment can be affected by your age.

Elderly cardio exercise equipment needs to be safe and with little risk of injury. The treadmill is great exercise equipment, since it's all about walking which is pretty natural to us. It does not create too much pressure on the joints but still burns enough calories while helping the lungs and the heart. Treadmill can still offer an intense workout for seniors without pressuring the ankles, hips and knees.

Aside from treadmills, recumbent cycles are another favorite among seniors. Recumbent cycles provide more comfortable and larger seat than stationary bikes. They also have a backrest offering more back support than traditional upright stationary bikes.

These bikes are easy to mount on, since they are lower to the ground. The bike or the user can simply sit down and start pedalling. The recumbent cycle can be used when rehabilitating from an injury. It does not only work on the lower body, but there are also models that incorporate upper body exercises.

There are also cushioned step machines which lessens the impact of the foot when stepping on the metal or on the floor. This equipment is popularly used by seniors in aerobic classes. It could also be used while watching television in the comfort of their homes.

Strengthening exercises would help build muscles and bones. However, they should be milder than the usual strengthening exercises performed. Muscles and the joints could be overstressed and lead to serious injury. Remember that as we grow older, our body's ability to recuperate is slower. A minor sprain could be troublesome for a couple of months, so taking it slow and easy is crucial.

Resistance band exercises are gaining popularity among seniors. They can help strengthen muscles and bones without too much risk of getting injured. They can be easily purchased in sports utility shops and have different tension levels.

There are some questions that could help you identify if the equipment you are considering to buy would benefit the elderly.

• Is the fitness equipment safe for the elderly and those who do not have enough experience?

• Is the fitness equipment safe and easy enough not to require full time spotting or a personal trainer?

• Is it easy to adjust to fit into the individual's ability?

• Will it make the user feel invigorated from an exercise and not exhausted?

Never forget to ask or consult your doctor, before purchasing any equipment. They could recommend an equipment that would suit your health and physical limitations. A cardio exercise equipment for the elderly should be comfortable, practical and at the same time leaves a feeling of being energized and exercised. When purchasing equipment, make sure that the elderly would actually be testing them. You could also read some reviews about the equipment to help you make right decision.

CHAPTER 7- CARDIO EXERCISE EQUIPMENT IN YOUR LIVING ROOM

Determining your goals would help you identify what equipment should be bought for the home gym.

Doing regular cardiovascular exercises has its numerous benefits. Aside from weight loss and prevention of diseases, it could also help in promoting overall health like better sleep, improved mood, less stress, etc. However, most of us have fast-paced lifestyle which makes it difficult to insert physical activity into our busy schedules. Having cardio exercise equipment at home could resolve that issue.

Signing up for an expensive gym membership may not be good idea if you are a person who dread walking to a room full of people and wait for you turn on the next machine. Aside from that, some people just do not have enough time to drive themselves to the gym.

Working out within the comfort of your home is getting popular over the years. In fact, in 2000 about $6.7 billion were spent on fitness equipment. The popularity of purchasing personal exercise equipment is increasing, making it possible for homeowners to find low-cost cardio exercise equipment without sacrificing the quality.

Generally, there are several questions that would be able to help you set-up your home gym.

• What are your goals in setting up your home gym?

• How much space would you need to setup your equipment?

• Are you the only one who would be working out? How many people would be using the gym?

• How much are you willing to spend on the equipment?

Determining your goals would help you identify what equipment will be purchased. For example, if you are after total cardio workout, then definitely a treadmill, elliptical, or stationary bike is needed. If you plan on building more muscle, then you would probably need pull-up bars, push-up stands, weights, etc.

Once you have decided to set-up a home gym, then you should consider where in the house you could set it up. You need to consider the space, since there are cardio equipment which cover a lot of space, like treadmills or the stationary step climber. The good news is that there are exercise equipment which can be folded or stored easily.

The home gym should also be in a room where it is properly ventilated and with enough sunlight. Working out in a dark room is never inviting. You would like to have your home gym look engaging, keep it organized and functional. Keep towels in the room. Make sure that there are water bottles in the room making it convenient for you to get a drink after a workout.

Cardio exercise equipment are mostly stationary equipment. For example, if you are on your stationary bike, then you will be pumping those pedals for the next half hour. Boredom is one reason why people stop working out. You could have a television in your home gym, so you could still catch up with favorite shows while sweating it out.

Setting up a home gym is not just about working out. You would also need to consider maintenance of your equipment. Not taking good care of them could cause you problems or worse, accidents.

Be cautious when using them. Don't just drop weights or shove things around. When storing you equipment, make sure that they are not exposed to excessive sunlight, dampness or other factors which may damage the equipment.

Chapter 8- Cardio Exercise Equipment on Wheels

Riding a bike, stationary or mobile is a great way to get a full cardio workout.

Biking is a good way to obtain an overall exercise. You get to undergo toning and cardio sessions. But there are times when the equipment falters and your busy schedule won't allow you to have an enjoying ride. Fortunately you can acquire an alternative.

All you need is to place a stationary bike in your favorite spot and voila you're all set. But unlike the normal bike that riders use you do not actually move from your original position. This bike is constructed with a solid back inverted T-frame attached firmly to the ground. The front wheel is hanging some inches off the floor so that you can freely move the pedals.

This workout machine is designed to provide a low impact workout. It has been tagged as one of the best cardio equipment which can also be effective in strengthening and toning the lower body. It is the smart choice for individuals with knee injuries undergoing therapy since knee muscles are conditioned without pressuring the joints.

It is recommended that you spend thirty minutes on the stationary bike in order to meet the ideal cardio requirements on a daily basis. For each session you have the option of adjusting the tension settings. These settings are similar with the gears found in regular bikes and can be used to increase the level of your workout.

There are two types from which you can choose namely upright and recumbent. For an upright model, you are seated just as you would on a standard bike. While some prefer this, there are others who complain of too much pressure on the groin and lower back even if these individuals have only spent a short time on the bike.

This flaw of the upright model paved the way for the creation of the recumbent model. It is the common equipment for individuals plagued by lower back problems as well as chronic back pain. This bike follows the go-cart design which allows you to sit in a reclined position with the legs stretched out rather than extended downward. This model offers both comfort and more efficient buttocks workout as compared to its counterpart.

The adjustment of the bike's seat is significant in ensuring that an effective and safe workout is achieved. When the legs are fully extended the angle of the seat should facilitate for the knee of the extended leg to remain slightly bent. The motion should be kept at a smooth pace with good rhythm. You should set the resistance at a level that your lower extremity can handle. Handlebars should be oriented within easy access.

Stationary bikes offer little upper body training. In order to compensate there have been designs wherein the handlebars move up and back. There are other variations which move the exerciser up and down. Experts believe these alterations might cause some problems regarding knee and back strains.

In theory there is no machine that is 100 percent perfect. There are flaws therefore sessions spent in cardio exercise equipment are not really enough if you want to maximize your full potential. In this case, you can add weight training in your routine.

CHAPTER 9- CARDIO EXERCISE EQUIPMENT MAINTENANCE

To ensure optimum performance, exercise equipment ahs to be cleaned and maintained frequently.

Cardio exercise equipment helps us achieve significant results in improving our overall health which is why a lot of people are investing in gym memberships and purchasing fitness equipment. Cardio exercise equipment are no longer just fitness machines, it is now considered investments.

To protect our investments, it is important to perform basic maintenance. If neglected, the equipment's performance may be affected. When benefit from our exercise equipment, since we are able to fully use them. But inability to perform basic and regular upkeep could affect how we benefit from out exercise machines. Eventually, small problems would lead to major equipment failure. Maintenance is not that hard, it just a matter of allotting time in cleaning and protecting them against the elements.

Some people think that just because their equipment is working properly, it would last like that for a long time. On the outside it may look fine, but the interior of the machine may be starting to have small problems. For example, if equipment with springs are exposed to dampness, the springs may get rusty and may lose its ability to compress and bounce back. In worst cases, equipment problems or failure could happen in the middle of the workout, causing accidents.

Sometimes, it is not just failure to do regular maintenance that could affect the equipment's performance. After a workout or some heavy training, we just drop our equipment or just shove or kick it aside. This could also damage the equipment. it is important to handle our equipment properly. After each workout, it is also important to store the machine properly. Make sure that it is stored away from excessive sunlight or dampness.

When cleaning hand rails and the upholstery, you will just need a cleaning pad, cleaner or cleaning solution and a dry towel or paper towels. Wiping the surfaces with cleaning pads and a cleaning solution could remove sweat, water or juice spills, etc. After wiping them with the cleanser, dry it with a towel to remove dampness, before storage. Avoid using the cleaning solutions on the treadmill's belt since it could affect the lubrication of the machine.

Make sure that they are free of dust and dirt. Make sure that the floor or mat under the treadmill is cleaned and vacuumed regularly. The lubrication should be checked monthly, while the belt should be inspected for tension and tracking every six months. The same goes for elliptical trainers.

Your stationary bike should not be making any squeaking noise. If it does, then check the pedals and the pedal shaft. It should be lubricated every three to four months. All exercise equipment should be checked every two to three months for loose nuts and bolts.

What most people forget is that the equipment manual is not only a guide for setting up the exercise machine. It also includes approved manufacturer methods of cleaning your exercise machine. Read and follow the instructions in the manual.

It is not only the mechanical equipment which needs to be checked. Other cardio exercise equipment should be cleaned, like the dumbbells and other weights. Maintenance could be easy as long as your make time for it. You could have a checklist on your

Barry Cromer

workout area where you have indicated the maintenance calendar for your machines.

CHAPTER 10- CARDIO EXERCISE EQUIPMENT

It is best to look at all the types of cardio equipment available before making a decision on which options are best.

Cardiovascular exercises are among the most popular routines known to fitness buffs. Not surprisingly, cardio exercise equipment are among the most well-known exercise machines. When you go to the gym, you could be 100% sure that you would be able to find cardio exercise equipment in many forms. In fact, in many fitness centers, such machines comprise of more than 50% of all available workout tools.

How many cardio exercise equipment do you know? This could be an interesting question. You might be surprised that you could know more than you thought. There are just too many of such machines, but of course you may not know all of them. It is said that every month, there is a new variation or evolution of current cardio exercise machines. Thus, there could be numerous of them by now. Here are the ones you could easily find.

The treadmill burns the greatest amount of calories compared to other cardio exercise equipment around. Simply by walking briskly, you could already burn up to 100 calories per mile. What's more ideal about this tool is that the speed could be adjusted to various levels for better outcomes.

Elliptical machines facilitate elliptical motions. Most compare the use of this cardio exercise equipment to actual cycling. Stand correctly on the foot pedals and move in an elliptical motion upon pedaling. Many experts assert that elliptical machines are more effective than other cardio exercise equipment in burning up more

Barry Cromer

calories. It is important to observe the proper and correct use of this product.

Stationary bikes are less intense in terms of calorie burning compared to other cardio exercise equipment. You would have to pedal up to four miles just to burn about a hundred calories. Stationary bikes could be less effective than treadmills but many people prefer to use them because they are fun and exciting.

Rowing machines are exercise machines that target the arms, the abdomen, the leg muscles, and the back. The indoor equipment are used like actual rowing boats. You need to sit stretched on the allocated machine seat. Use the machine correctly or under the appropriate supervision of a personal fitness trainer for best results.

The recumbent bike could burn more calories than everyone's favorite, the treadmill. However, it could burn less calories compared to the elliptical machine. This machine is not the type that experts usually recommend to people who need to shed off more than 30 pounds of excessive weight.

Tread climbers are among the newest cardio exercise machines in the market. They could be considered as the best cardio exercise. Needless to say, tread climbers are combining the wonders of a treadmill and climbing equipment. You could not run on this one. You could only walk. However, the calories burned are much greater.

Swing machines usually are considered as passive cardio exercise equipment. This cardio exercise equipment is rare because it is among the very few that requires the user to lie down to the floor while executing the exercise. Its effectiveness could never be underestimated, though.

Chapter 11- Carefree Cardio Exercise Equipment

Treadmills are great for persons that live in areas that tend are prone to inclement weather. There is no excuse for not exercising.

The heart plays the vital role of pumping blood throughout the body. That is why it should be properly cared for. One very good way to do so is through exercise. Let's take a look at one of the cardio equipment that allows you to perform your routines anytime of the day within the comforts of your home.

So you plan to take a jog or even just a walk but the weather won't allow you to do so. It's a good thing you have the option of owning a treadmill. It is a low impact cardio machine that paves the way for walking, jogging, and even running in place. This is made possible by a moving belt situated over a deck.

You can choose between a manual and a motorized treadmill. The manual type is lighter and less expensive. You can easily fold it away, slide it under your bed or put it inside your closet. The running belt is wrapped around rollers giving way for a raised deck.

As you begin to walk on the belt your actual weight produces friction that is necessary for your feet to move the belt over the rollers. The belt turns underneath you as you walk in place. There are provided side rails which you can use for safety support. At the front portion of the treadmill you will find a console that serves as support for both the walking platform and side rails.

The motorized form is of course heavier, less portable, and can make you spend more. But then again it can provide a much more satisfying workout experience. The running belt is being operated by a self-powered motor that is situated beneath your feet. The trifecta of walking, jogging, and running is allowed since the speed of the machine can be adjusted. In this type make sure you warm-up properly before going to higher speeds.

Treadmills can come with a lot of features. Generally speaking the more expensive a machine is the more features it has to offer. You can have preconfigured programs that suit your body's present condition and capacity. There are different difficulty levels that are fit for the greenhorn up to the more advanced runner.

Speed variations are not the only ones that can be manipulated during a workout session. You can also alter the condition of the deck. The deck of a motorized treadmill can be tilted just like the conditions of tricky uphill surfaces and terrains. It's up to your preference when it comes to how inclined your exercise experience will be.

The present batch of treadmills normally come with an electronic heart rate monitor which will allow you to determine if you are progressing well enough towards your desired workout. Chest-wrap monitors are usually favored over the ear clip type. The wireless variation of the chest-wrap comes with an alarm that notifies you when your heart rate is way below or above your acceptable range.

In the near future cardio exercise equipment like the treadmill will be enhanced by technology. Virtual reality will be incorporated in the features of the machine. You are now one button away from walking, jogging, or running on any part of the planet.

CHAPTER 12- CHECKLIST BEFORE BUYING CARDIO EXERCISE EQUIPMENT

Before you go shopping, think of the exercises you want to do to succeed in your fitness goal.

People exercise for four basic reasons: to increase cardiovascular endurance, muscle strength, muscle endurance, and flexibility. If you're a person whose goal is to increase cardiovascular endurance, you need to do workouts which will strengthen your heart and enhance your metabolism. Examples of these workouts are walking, jogging, running and cross training. These can be done outdoors or indoors.

To maintain the habit of regular exercise, it is advised to use cardio exercise equipment. You can access various types of this equipment at fitness gyms. However, if you think you can stick to your workout more by having a home gym, there are wide varieties of affordable equipment you can invest. Here are the things you need to consider before buying cardio exercise equipment:

1. Activities you want to do - Before you go shopping, think of the exercises you want to do to succeed in your fitness goal. If you prefer walking, jogging and running, treadmill is perfect for you. If you prefer cross-country skiing, you may try elliptical trainers. If you prefer cycling and want to be more comfortable while doing a workout, a stationary bike is for you.

2. Space - Some cardio exercise equipment that can be folded so you can save storage space. Good examples of this are treadmills. Fitness experts recommend folding treadmills than non-folding treadmills as they are easy to keep. However, folding treadmills are more expensive that their non-folding counterparts. Equipment

that requires larger space is elliptical trainers. This machine gives you the advantage of upper and lower body workout which is an excellent overall exercise.

The least equipment that requires space is the stationary bikes. It is also easy to read magazines, books, watch TV while using the stationary bikes. If you prefer doing other stuffs like the ones mentioned, stationary bike is the right equipment for you.

3. Reviews - It is always best to read consumer reviews before finally deciding to buy cardio exercise equipment. You can check reviews through the internet; websites like askthetrainer.com and homegymsadviser.com offer tips, reviews and fitness guides. You can also refer to fitness books like "The Men's Health Home Workout Bible, Fitness for Life, and the Woman's Workout Bible.

4. Budget - You need to determine what cardio exercise equipment you exactly want to get the best of what you pay for. Fitness experts recommend choosing brands that are a little expensive but of high-quality rather than the cheap ones. Cheaper brands are usually mass-produced. If you intend to buy a treadmill just for walking, you can already buy a good quality and durable treadmill at the cost of $1,000. If you're a runner, best buy items usually rangers from $1,500 - $2,000. Fitness experts recommend to buy elliptical trainers costing more than $1,000 as cheaper machines can only hold up to light use.

There are two main types of cardio exercise bikes: the recumbent and the upright. You can already buy a good quality bike at the cost of $450. Expensive brands of bikes cost above $1,390 while the cheapest cost below $170. Common problems among cheaper brands of bikes include missing parts, difficult to assembly, and damage to brittle or plastic parts during shipping.

CHAPTER 13- CHOOSING CARDIO EXERCISE EQUIPMENT

As soon as you have a plan in place you can start shopping for exercise equipment. Once you have determined what exercise equipment you prefer, then you could start scouting for prices.

Cardiovascular exercises boost your overall system, the heart and lungs become stronger; muscles and joints are nourished, strengthened, and is improved with their mobility. More and more people are now beginning to understand the importance of regular exercise and activity. In fact, in 2006 Club Industry's Fitness Business Pro Purchasing Power Survey, about 55% of the respondents included cardio exercise equipment in their shopping list.

If you are planning to purchase a cardio exercise equipment, here are some useful tips that could help you choose the right one.

• Identify what cardio machine you would like to have.

There are numerous types of cardio equipment on the market, if you walked into a fitness equipment store, you could get overwhelmed with the different equipment and various models. Trainers, family members or your partner may recommend different kinds of equipment. But it is important to consider what cardio machine you would like to have. You will be using that equipment every day for a long time, so it pays to get a machine that you actually like and would be using every day.

• Consider your budget.

Barry Cromer

Once you have determined what exercise equipment you prefer, then you could start scouting for prices. There is nothing wrong with shopping around. You could check the running price for both brand-new and pre-owned exercise equipment. Pre-owned are less expensive, just be sure that they are in good condition. To give you an idea, treadmills and stationary bikes had a price range of $200 to $3,000, depending on its features. You could also check websites for their prices.

• Scouting for places to buy equipment.

There are local sporting and fitness stores that sell exercise equipment. The internet is also a rich source of information. Don't just check one website and stick with it. Online shops are becoming so competitive; prices tend to be lower than actual fitness stores. If you have decided to purchase from an online store, then you would need to consider about the shipping cost, warranties and of course, service agreements.

• Check the warranty and return policy.

When making the purchase from online stores always look for the warranty and return policy. When the equipment is shipped, it is not impossible that the equipment would incur damages while being transported.

• Other factors.

If you have already decided on the exercise equipment, model and price range, then you would have to consider the physical and mechanical aspects of the machine. For example whether you are buying pre-owned equipment or brand-new ones, check the motor, intensity and resistance levels of the workout, and if you would be able to take advantage of these. Take a look if the machine's motor will be operating smoothly.

Exercise Equipment: Selecting the Best for Cardio Workouts
Yearly, Americans would spend millions of dollars in purchasing cardio exercise equipment which is sometimes used or just placed in the corner to gather dust just because they are the wrong equipment for you. Consider purchasing cardio exercise equipment as a form of investment. Not only are you investing on property, but also on your health and overall well-being..

CHAPTER 14- FINDING THE BEST CARDIO EXERCISE EQUIPMENT FOR YOURSELF

If you are not sure of the types of exercise equipment to purchase for your home gym consult with an fitness professional.

Do you plan to embark on a heavy cardiovascular program to help your body lose excessive weight? You are on the right track. Cardiovascular exercises help accelerate the body's metabolism so that stored fats and calories would be burned. To achieve your cardiovascular goals, you could use cardio exercise equipment. There are many of such machines that are sold commercially these days. How could you find the best one for your own training? It could be an exhilarating task but you could be guided accordingly by these simple insights.

First, always remember that what could be the best cardio exercise machine for your friend may not be the best for you. This is because your body is naturally different compared to the body of your friend. The most significant goal of a good cardiovascular exercise is increasing your heart rate. This way, more blood could be pumped into the heart. More calories would be burned, as indicated by the excessive sweat your body produce. You could help yourself raise the rate of your heartbeat even without the use of a machine. But for best results and to stave off possible idling, investing in cardio exercise equipment would be advisable.

The decision about the best cardio exercise equipment could primarily depend on several important factors. First, the machine may be fun or not. It could seem very amateurish to seek enjoyment and excitement when doing cardio exercise. But if it works, why should you divert from the strategy? If you truly enjoy a particular cardio exercise machine, you surely would be more motivated to use it. If you hate it, you may notice that you are actually holding back yourself from using it. Thus, you would get no actual benefit from not using the best cardio exercise machine.

Second, the exercise machine should not exacerbate any physical discomfort or problem. Everything should be taken in moderation. The statement is applicable in the use of cardio exercise equipment. If you are performing a single motion for numerous times in hours, you would definitely achieve muscle imbalances. This would lead to dynamic and static problems regarding your posture. Thus, if you are sitting all day in your job, the popular stationary bike is absolutely not the best cardio exercise machine for you. In the same way, bad knee condition should prevent you from using the stair master machine.

Is the cardio exercise equipment consistent and aligned with your personal goals? If you are aiming to burn fat, maintain fitness of heart, and improve weight, cardio machines are the right exercise tools to use. If your goals are focused on improving performance, cardio exercise machines that are most closely related to any given activity are appropriate. If you want to improve your performance as a marathon runner, you should choose the treadmill.

It would help improve your running. It does not mean that you should refrain from using the stationary bike as frequently as you like, though.

CHAPTER 15- GETTING BACK TO BASICS-EXERCISE EQUIPMENT

You should not be too hasty in judging new and innovative cardio exercise equipment

Admit it or not you have become one of those people who have turned away from an unhealthy lifestyle. Like many individuals at present you have become health conscious especially when it comes to cardio issues. You look forward into being acquainted with reliable exercise equipment.

You might not know it but a rowing machine exists. It is usually one of the most neglected contraptions in the gym because people are a bit ignorant on how it should be properly used. This machine is designed to simulate rowing motions. You have to understand that it is not built for resistance exercises. People who utilize it often pull very hard resulting into bad form and ineffective workout.

The core principle in using a rowing machine is motivation. In order to maximize its full benefits you have to intensify the speed of your workouts. You have absolute control. Only you can dictate where a single session can go.

The arc trainer is one of the newest brands of non-impact cardio equipment that is steadily gaining popularity within the circles of gym-goers. It consists of two platforms that allow you to swing your legs back and forth. You can adjust the speed and resistance to modify the scissor-like movements of your legs thus intensifying your cardio session.

Non-impact machines are the ideal forms of cardio equipment specifically for persons suffering from chronic joint problems. The arc trainer can increase you heart rate without putting too much pressure on your lower extremities but don't let the non-impact nature of the machine compromise each workout. Make sure that your heart rate is maintained within high levels based on your target parameter.

Another one of the newest types of cardio equipment situated on the forgotten zone of local gyms is the Versa climber. But this should not be the case since this machine is effective in cardio conditioning. It demands that you climb vertically directly opposing the force of gravity. Both your upper and lower body is active thus you heart rate spikes up in a swift manner.

The machine can be very challenging especially when you increase the resistance. With each push and pull you're assured that your muscles are performing. The Versa climber is a cardio contraption that can be utilized for interval training. You can have a tough five minutes on the machine given normal intensity levels. Thus it would be advisable to alternately do your workout with another cardio machine like the stationary bike wherein you have the luxury of making a quick transition.

Hand ergometers or hand bikes are the ones being used by individuals undergoing rehabilitation because of a fractured leg or sprained ankle. Your heart rate goes up quickly when using these machines as compared to the leg cardio equipment. This is because your arms are closer to your heart. Since a session on this contraption can be a bit boring you might want to listen to your favorite tunes.

You should not be too hasty in judging new and innovative cardio exercise equipment. Yes the conventional ones are tried and tested but the other machines in your local gym were placed there for a reason. Do not neglect them. Give them a try and you will see that they are just as effective as the traditional treadmills and stationary bikes.

CHAPTER 16- INSIGHT ON CARDIO EXERCISE EQUIPMENT

Never purchase a machine just because it is popular, you will never use it. Only get what is necessary and what you will actually use.

You always find yourself standing in a room full of different cardiovascular machines at the gym. There are just too many of them: treadmills, stair steppers, elliptical machines, stationary bikes, and rowing machines. If you are finding it hard to decide which to use in the gym, it surely would be harder to make up your mind about which cardio exercise equipment to choose and buy for your use at home.

Ask yourself: which cardio exercise machine to use: the one that brings the most fit, the tool that burns the greatest amount of calories, or the equipment that brings about least impact on your own joints? All these are of course valid concerns that you should not be neglecting. Bryant A. Stamford, an exercise physiologist, asserts that none of the questions could be considered as the most important to ask yourself. Instead, one good and logical question you should ask yourself is: 'Which cardio exercise machine do you truly want to use?'

When it comes to weight management and exercise training, the usual case is that someone who desperately needs to shed off excess weight is usually the one who is easily turned off by any cardio exercise. Many experts argue that it is the worst to mold anyone into accepting an exercise program that other people say is the best. To make the most of any cardio exercise program, you need to know what is good for you, not what is good for other people. Surely, the best cardio exercise equipment for your neighbor is not as effective to you.

Instead of quickly choosing elliptical trainer that your friend recommended or the popular treadmill specifically for its calorie-burning factor, you should first and foremost figure out and identify the exercise machine that truly feels best to you. Everything else should be secondary. In other words, the best and most effective piece of all exercise equipment is that which you are most willing to regularly use. It would not make sense choosing a machine that you do not feel like using every day. You have to exude a genuine interest on the equipment.

How could you determine the best cardio exercise equipment that is best for you? You may jumpstart on your decision-making process by taking the choice while you are at the gym. The venue surely is complete with all the necessary and important cardio exercise machines. Take time to try out each of the equipment. This way, you could easily identify which one is the most effective and most comfortable for you.

Prioritize comfort. It is important that you find cardio exercise equipment that you are enjoying to use. You would not enjoy using a machine if it does not feel comfortable using it. Thus, the best cardio exercise machine is the one that you certainly would use. It is not the equipment that is most popular in the market or that which is recommended by your peers. It is what your body wants to use.

CHAPTER 17- LOOKING FOR CARDIO EXERCISE EQUIPMENT

It will take time to find the perfect set of cardio exercise equipment so do not worry if you cannot find what you want on the first attempt.

Healthy body and mind is important for achieving a healthier and more productive life. Cardiovascular exercises are exercise routines that are designed specifically to help the body accelerate its metabolism and burn up more calories. The routines could help you bolster blood flow as well as heart rate. Ultimately, they could even help keep the body in ideal shape. If you are aiming to perform aerobic tasks better and more correctly, you should instead opt to use specific cardio exercise equipment.

Two of the most popular and sought-after cardio exercise equipment is of course the treadmill and the stationary bike. It is not surprising that they are considered as staples or must-haves in every gym. Such machines are now easier to find and are practical to use. Owning such tools would enable you to perform cardiovascular exercises at home. In general, the more you sweat; the better is the outcome to your overall health.

There are other popular forms of cardio exercise equipment available. It is time you take a closer look at the most sough-after. Treadmills are facilitating walking, running, and jogging indoors. You could adjust the speed depending on your purpose. These machines have timers and are usually featuring built-in calorie calculators. The treadmill could stimulate and use almost every muscle in your body. It is ideal for trimming down tummy bulges.

The stationary bike is another popular cardio exercise machine. It is best for people suffering from arthritis and for those who could not use the treadmill. By adding resistance to the bike, you could significantly strengthen muscles in your legs. In the long run, the use of the machine could help you improve your overall stamina.

Swing machines usually are considered as passive cardio exercise equipment. To use the tool, lie down flat to the floor. Keep your feet along the groves of the machines or at the footrest. You may adjust the speed and at the same time set the timer. In no time, the footrest would swing back and then forth to carry your feet in identical motions. The movement should be carried throughout the body. Relax and breathe very deeply so you could achieve an ideal workout experience.

Rowing machines are exercise machines that target the arms, the abdomen, the leg muscles, and the back. The indoor equipment are used like actual rowing boats. You need to sit stretched on the allocated machine seat. Use the machine correctly or under the appropriate supervision of a personal fitness trainer for best results. Be cautious when using the machine because wrong form in using it could lead to uncomfortable body strains.

Elliptical machines facilitate elliptical motions. Most compare the use of this cardio exercise equipment to actual cycling. Stand correctly on the foot pedals and move in an elliptical motion upon pedaling. Many experts assert that elliptical machines are more effective than other cardio exercise equipment in burning up more calories. It is important to observe the proper and correct use of this product.

CHAPTER 18- POPULAR CARDIO EXERCISE EQUIPMENT

Each type of cardio exercise equipment can help you to achieve varying degrees of a workout. It is best to choose one that will provide a challenge for a while.

Are you considering buying and using particular cardiovascular exercise machines? You should be aware that there are just too many of them. You could not possibly choose, buy, and use all. It would be appropriate if you choose one and decide to use it regularly. To be able to make the best choice, it would be helpful if you would know what to expect from several of the most popular cardio exercise equipment available.

The treadmill

This machine burns the greatest amount of calories compared to other cardio exercise equipment around. Simply by walking briskly, you could already burn up to 100 calories per mile. What's more ideal about this tool is that the speed could be adjusted to various levels for better outcomes. One setback is that heavy use of treadmill could bring about unlikely pain or discomfort in your lower back or knees.

Stair steppers and elliptical machines

This equipment could serve as good alternatives to the popular treadmill. Because you are using them while in a standing position, you would be prompted to use more muscle mass. This way, the rate or calorie burning could remain high. Elliptical machines with added arm components could help burn much more calories. The setback is that these machines could pose unlikely impact to the joints.

Stationary bikes

These machines are simply described as less intense in terms of calorie burning compared to other cardio exercise equipment. You would have to pedal up to four miles just to burn about a hundred calories. Stationary bikes could be less effective than treadmills but many people prefer to use them because they are fun and exciting. The common setback to the use of these bikes is that there could be possible knee strain.

Rowing machine

Many people are misled about how a rowing machine really works. The usual misconception is that the tool is primarily designed to facilitate an upper-body workout. In reality, rowing machines are actually advanced cardiovascular exercise machines. You would be required to use more muscle groups. Hence, you could burn more calories. The common setback is that extra weight brings about back pain. There could even be muscle spasms on the upper-body area.

Versa climbers

These cardio exercise equipment are among the best and most effective cardiovascular machines available. The tool is designed in a way that would facilitate you to take a movement as if you are climbing vertically. Your body would be prompted to work against gravity. Thus, there is more work and more calories are burned. By using the lower and upper bodies equally, you could significantly boost your heart rate very quickly.

Exercise Equipment: Selecting the Best for Cardio Workouts
Have you made up your mind? Which of the above-mentioned cardio exercise equipment would be best for you? You have to make the decision on your own. You would be the one using the machine. You need not depend on what your doctor, friends, or colleagues would recommend. Make the best and wisest choice now.

Chapter 19- Revving Up With Cardio Exercise Equipment

Remember that cardio exercises speed up the heart rate so you have to monitor yourself to ensure it is not being overdone.

Simple exercises can be done to boost your cardio conditioning. You can jog in the park every morning. You can take the stairs instead of using the elevator. But if you choose to heighten each training session so as to maximize your full potential then you need to get the proper equipment.

One device that can target your heart's performance is the stair climber. It is a machine that provides the resistance and conditioning you can attain by completing a flight of stairs. It is commonly paired up with aerobic routines especially when the venue does not provide the appropriate set of stairs.

The first kind of this machine entered the fitness scenario in 1983 via the famed Stairmaster model. It was built having a pair of pedals which you can utilize in order to stand straight. It is equipped with handlebars which can provide additional support and balance.

The important concept when using this machine is to never put too much weight on the handlebars. By doing so, you do not adhere to the standard form of the workout. Moreover, you become susceptible to wrist injuries. You should also maintain proper body alignment and positioning particularly on the knees in order to prevent any sort of straining and injury.

You are given the chance to manipulate the level of your workout by adjusting the resistance and speed. This feature is present on the various types of the stair climber. The version which is cylinder driven comes in a less expensive price. In this version resistance is produced via hydraulic fluid or air and a knob is turned to adjust the resistance level. Models that are more expensive are computer-controlled and have additional features like preconfigured workout programs and analysis indicating the calories burned along with your heart rate.

Although the main function of the stair climber is to provide adequate cardio training it can also lead the way for the conditioning of the muscles in the thighs, buttocks, and calves. You can further increase the toning capacities of this device by incorporating the use of ankle weight during your sessions. As you progress with your routines and you think you've achieved proper balancing you can gradually let go of the handlebars.

Treadmills are the common machines used to increase the heart's performance but if you have undergone any trauma or injury on the joints of your lower extremity then chances are you won't be able to handle the impact. In this case the elliptical trainer may help you get through the rehabilitation period while maintaining the appropriate workout for your heart. Plus you get to burn the same calories with a less effort on your part.

Elliptical trainer machines offer other features that may not be present in common treadmills. It allows you to exercise in the normal forward motion but can also present routines in a reverse direction. The change of direction will give you the chance to target various sets of muscles thus your workout is revved up to higher levels.

You can choose from a wide array of cardio exercise equipment but you have to realize that each session does not only aim to strengthen the targeted body part. Each anatomical area should be kept in good condition and within normal functioning levels.

Barry Cromer

Chapter 20- Save When Buying Cardio Exercise Equipment

When buying exercise equipment, budget has to be taken into consideration. Don't go over budget but buy the best that you can afford.

It pays to stay really fit and healthy. You must regularly go to the gym to workout and do rigorous cardiovascular exercises. But unfortunately, you may not always find time to do so. That is why knowing how to save in buying good cardio exercise equipment will be of great help to you.

If you aim to keep your weight controlled, you need to exercise regularly. You need to make use of specific cardio gym equipment for the appropriate exercise program for you. You need to sweat and improve your heart's overall health. Cardio exercises can also help maintain circulatory health.

Because you will not always have the convenient and spare time to spend in going to the gym, you need to invest in buying some useful cardio exercise equipment for your home. Yes, you may not need to buy all the equipment you see in your gym. But you can buy those that are really needed.

If you are aiming to buy your own cardio exercise equipment for home use, you need to do so wisely. There are several impediments that will prevent you from buying machines that you can do without. One is sufficient space at home.

You do not need to abruptly convert your home into a gym in an instant. There are still more important things and items that should be prioritized within your house.

Another factor will be the more important and obvious---costs. You need to save money for many other important purposes. That is because it is not that easy to earn a living nowadays. You need to be extra wise when spending your money down to the last cent.

Here are some useful tips when you aim to save money in buying cardio exercise equipment:

• Take time to plan cardio exercises you will do and where you will put your exercise equipment. Consider the space available. You do not need equipment that will only be left non-useful in the garage or elsewhere because the allotted space inside the house will not be able to accommodate all the equipment. Tread mills for example take a lot of space.

• Know what cardio exercise equipment you need and which ones you can easily install and use at home. You might need opinion or recommendation from your gym instructor for a partial list of must-buy exercise equipment for your home.

• Compare before you shop. Just like when shopping or buying anything from the department store or from the retail shop, you may need to look at and compare price tags before you finally make the acquisition.

• Ask peers and other experts about which exercise equipment to buy. Know which brands will be ideal and which equipment will be cheaper compared to others. Also seek for feedbacks and experiences about each machine. By doing so, you can avoid committing the same mistakes done by your friends when they purchased their own cardio exercise equipment.

• You can buy cardio exercise equipment and other fitness machines one by one. Buying a number of equipment all at the same time can be very hard on the pocket. Buying equipment one by one is by far like buying merchandise on an installment basis.

CHAPTER 21- THE BEST CARDIO EXERCISE EQUIPMENT AVAILABLE

Shopping for exercise equipment can be challenging so it is best to narrow it down by brand, price range and function to make the selection process less stressful.

What is the best cardiovascular exercise machine available in the market today? Answering this question could be exhilarating and disappointing at the same time. It is because there are just too many cardio exercise equipment commercially out in the market. You surely would be overwhelmed and excited if you would look and try out each of the equipment. Every machine is sophisticated, fashionable, and fun. There are even various brands, each offering different and breakthrough features to outpace and outshine one another.

If you would ask the experts, the best cardio exercise machine would be the one for fat loss. Its functionality and effectiveness would depend on your current shape and weight. Usually, people who aim to lose more than 30 pounds are advised to start by using the popular treadmill. Choose the machine without incline then set a comfortable speed. You could increase it as fat weight is trimmed and cardiovascular efficiency is improved. You could challenge your system by increasing your speed effectively. Eventually, as you go on, you could use the incline function of the treadmill. Doing so would be best if you want to take off those bulges in the hamstring area.

For people who target losing less than 30 pounds, experts usually recommend the cross trainer elliptical machine. This cardio exercise machine is the one that enables movement of the arms. This is also recommended to advanced bodybuilders. Cross trainer elliptical machine stimulates the body's running motion. However, as it does so, the impact on the ankles and knees are lessened, if not totally eliminated. Results brought about by this particular machine are usually fast because the calories are quickly and effectively burned throughout the duration of the entire activity. Using the machine could burn more stored calories than what the regular treadmill could do.

The recumbent bike should never be overlooked. The equipment could facilitate a very effective cardio workout especially when tension is set to impact the knees. In comparison, the recumbent bike could burn more calories than everyone's favorite, the treadmill. However, it could burn less calories compared to the elliptical machine. This machine is not the type that experts usually recommend to people who need to shed off more than 30 pounds of excessive weight. Some users attest that using this one is so much fun. It makes the body active and hyper.

Lastly, you may consider the stairstepper. It is a middle-of-the-road choice for people who need to lose less than 30 pounds. However, like most users, you may not completely like the motion involved. This is the type of cardio exercise equipment that you would only prefer to use if there is no other option available. You may notice that not many people use it in the gym. But regardless of its likability, the stairstepper is effective in trimming excess body weight.

You need to use it at a steady tempo within just about 20 minutes to 45 minutes on a daily basis for best results. There is no more need to set high resistance.

CHAPTER 22- TIPS FOR BUYING HOME CARDIO EXERCISE EQUIPMENT

The main tips to bear in mind when buying exercise equipment is to write down what you are looking for beforehand as you can get distracted in the store and end up purchasing what you really do not need.

Buying exercise equipment for your home is a great way to save money in doing physical training to increase your heart health. However, there are few things to consider like space availability, power source and budget. The following are helpful tips for you to choose the best cardio exercise equipment or equipment for your home gym.

1. Stick with the basics - It's normal to feel overwhelmed but in choosing exercise equipment, you should limit your choice to machines that mimic real life movements like treadmill or stationary bikes.

2. Size up your space - If you have a very limited space, it is best to consider equipment that fits easily into tight quarters like an exercise bike. Some machines can be folded for better and compact storage but do you have a clear area to use them?

3. Consider the location - If you prefer watching TV while doing cardio exercises, add at least another 8 feet in your space estimate.

4. Try only the ones that interest you - Ok, so you're excited to set up your home gym, however, you need to do trial exercises first. You can do this by getting a membership at a nearby gym. Familiarize yourself with different machines. The home versions of the machines you can see at fitness gyms may be a bit smaller and

less durable but trying them on will give you an idea of what you need you most.

5. Consider your health background - If you had injuries before never try stair climbers. If you have bad back stay away from rowers and cross-country ski machines. Do not buy exercise equipment that will only complicate your previous injuries.

6. Look for safety features - Consider buying cardio exercise equipment with safety features especially if you have kids at home.

7. Ask for family member's preference - Since you'll be setting up your cardio exercise equipment at home, some family members might also be interested in using it. Ask for the opinion of your family members for a more fun and motivating physical training.

8. Consider your fitness level - Choose a cardio exercise equipment that is both enjoyable and challenging for you. Exercise bikes and skiing type machines are good in improving your aerobic fitness.

9. Quality first - Remember, if one product is sold at lower prices, chances are, it's mass produced and of low quality. Generally, you get what you pay for. So, you should not always believe everything you see on infomercials as some of these tend to be deceiving.

10. Consult to your doctor - Ask first your physician or orthopedist before buying cardio exercise equipment. Having an injury or medical condition would affect your physical training. However, that does not mean you have to curtail your training. Physical activity is sometimes better to inactivity when you are rehabilitating from an injury. For example: people with injured or subpar knees can still ride a stationary bike or people with lower back pain can still train effectively, provided they do the correct strengthening exercises.

Chapter 23- Tips When Buying Cardio Exercise Equipment

Set realistic goals. Before you buy any of the available cardio exercise equipment, you should have already set your weight loss targets.

If you intend to lose weight, you should prefer cardiovascular exercises. Thus, when investing in workout machines, it is a necessity to choose any of the available cardio exercise equipment. To be able to realize your fitness and weight loss goals, you need to work out smart. Choose and buy the best machine that you think would be most useful for your goals. Here are some guidelines.

Choose cardio exercise equipment that feels very right. Take note of the impact brought about by such machines. If you have lower back problems, it is definitely not a good idea to choose a stationary bicycle over a treadmill. Always bear in mind that in choosing and buying the tools, it should not be about the cardio exercise machine. Prioritize the relationship between your body and the equipment. If any part of your body hurts of gets uncomfortable when using a machine, ditch it.

Choose a machine that would facilitate use of more muscles. In general, more muscles used translate to more calories burned. However, be aware of the flipside of the coin. Using more muscles in cardio exercise equipment would quickly bring about fatigue, especially if you are a beginner. Take it slowly but surely.

Modify or vary your routine. Do not use the elliptical machine every day. You have to introduce variety so your muscles and yourself would not be bored. Experiment and try out different pre-programmed workouts. They could include variations in intensity and speed. Change the way you usually workout. You may use various cardio exercise equipment in a week for variety and challenge.

Be mindful of time. You could use time to get the most out of every cardio exercise machine. Before you do a workout, set a time for completing the routines. For instance, you may give yourself just about half an hour to complete the workout. Follow your schedule strictly. This way, you would be forced to make the most of available time.

Mix it up. Do not stay on a favorite cardio exercise machine. As mentioned, change your routine and use other machines to be able to overcome and prevent boredom. Adapt to the changes imposed. It is advisable not to do the same routines all the time.

Ignore readouts. It is hard to resist the temptation of monitoring how much calories you have burned up at the end of an exercise. Experts assert that it is not ideal to do this practice. Instead, take a cue on how you actually feel. Are you tired? Then you may need to slow down or stop. It is important not to overwork or exhaust yourself.

Lastly, set realistic goals. Before you buy any of the available cardio exercise equipment, you should have already set your weight loss targets. This way, you would be guided more appropriately about which machine to buy and use. It is important not to set impossible goals. Avoid disappointments. Set targets that are achievable and possible.

CHAPTER 24- TYPES OF CARDIO EXERCISE EQUIPMENT

Always do test runs before you buy exercise equipment. Try out all the features then make your decision

Cardiovascular exercises are activities which engage large muscle groups to exercises. These exercises are known to have an impact on a person's blood pressure, calorie burning and weight loss. To enhance its benefits, cardio exercise equipment can be used. Cardio exercise equipment makes it possible to engage in a workout even when living in a controlled space, like your home.

Since cardiovascular exercises aim to increase heart rate using large muscles, it is common to use leg muscles like in walking and running. To make the whole body moving, leg and arm movements are incorporated in the workout regime. There are different types of cardiovascular exercise equipment.

• Treadmill

There are studies showing that exercising in the treadmill is better than other fitness equipment since it is natural for people to walk and run. You could adjust it settings, allowing you to walk, jog or run even in your living room. There are automatic and manual treadmills which can be purchased based on the customer's preference. Aside from that, maintenance and storage is not that demanding. There are treadmills which can be bought for as much as $200.

• Stationary step machines

Exercise Equipment: Selecting the Best for Cardio Workouts

This exercise equipment burns calories big time, which makes it a fixture in most fitness gyms. It also helps in toning or enhancing hips, legs and butts. Stationary step machines or stair climbers would allow you to check how much calories you have burned when exercising.

Some people find this equipment to be the most difficult of all the cardio exercise equipment. They provide great workout for the lower body as long as you use it properly. It could cause problems on knees and feet if the weight and force are not used properly.

• Exercise stationary bikes

These are mounted bikes which are steadily attached on the ground. A great way to get a cardio workout at home, especially for beginners since it does need special skill to operate or use. There is also a smaller risk of injury. According to studies, about 30 minutes on the stationary bike would be enough.

They are also ideal if you have limited space. They are mobile and can be moved to different places of the house. There are also some bikes that do not need to be plugged into an outlet.

• Elliptical trainers

Along with treadmills, elliptical trainers are among the most popular cardio exercise equipment. The great thing about elliptical trainers is that there is little or no impact at all which makes it ideal for people who have been suffering from joint muscle. It proved to be a great exercise equipment for seniors and the elderly who have knee and joint problems.

• Rowing machines

They are not that popular compared to treadmills or elliptical trainers but they provide an overall and intense cardio workout. Rowing machines would sometimes include monitors that provide you information how much calories you are burning. They can also be folded and stored easily.

What makes cardio exercise equipment notable is that they provide better results, not only in enhancing your physical appearance but also in improving overall health. Before making any purchase, you could try cardio exercise equipment in a fitness gym to help you get an idea about the equipment and if you would be able to use it in the long run.

CHAPTER 25- WHAT TO LOOK FOR IN A CARDIO EXERCISE EQUIPMENT

Something to consider when purchasing exercise equipment is the warranty; always find that out before making the purchase

Whether you're going to purchase cardio exercise equipment for the first time or you're just going to add another piece to your home gym, it is important to do a little research before you finalize your decision. Here's a brief overview of the things you need to look for in cardio exercise equipment:

1. Quality - You essentially get what you pay for, that is why in making a purchase it is important to go for the quality more than anything else. You may be tempted to buy cheaper equipment but remember, most of them are mass - produced. For treadmills, among of the best picks are Landice L8 Treadmill, Landice L7 Treadmill, True Z5.0, Precor 9.35 Treadmill, Bodyguard 312C Treadmill, Nordic Track 8600, and Smooth 9.45 Treadmill. You should expect spending $3,000 up if you want to buy high quality treadmills.

Good quality elliptical trainers, on the other hand, usually cost more than $5,000, that is why you should be 100% sure in purchasing this exercise equipment. Among of the items that receive excellent consumer feedbacks are; Sole E55 Elliptical Trainer, Smooth 3.2 Elliptical Trainer, New Balance 9.0e Elliptical Trainer, and Spirit ZE110 Elliptical Trainer.

2. Uses - When you buy a machine, it is important to go for the item that you will most likely use. Don't get persuaded by commercials and limit your choices to the machine that mimic your most enjoyable physical trainings.

3. Machines that will fit in your space - If you have a limited space, it is best to choose a cardio exercise equipment that can be folded and fits easily into tight quarters like stationary bikes.

4. Items that respect your previous injuries or other health situations - Before buying a cardio exercise equipment, you will need to consult your physician first. If you have bad knees, you might not be allowed to use stair climbers. If you have bad back, you might not be allowed to use rowers and cross country ski machines.

5. Items with safety features - If you have kids at home, you should buy an equipment or equipment that are safeguarded.

6. Items that are challenging to you - Are you a beginner or are trying to achieve another fitness level? Don't buy an item whose exercises it allows are far less than or more than your current fitness level.

7. With 90 days warranty - When buying cardio exercise equipment, ask about warranty for parts and labor.

8. Items made of excellent materials - Always check if the cushioning and upholstery are in stellar condition. Compare the equipment with the ones you see in gym. Most home cardio exercise equipment is smaller versions of those available on gyms.

Refer on the following list to determine the best cardio exercise equipment for you. Contrary to what you hear, no cardio equipment is really better than the other. Which means that the success of your cardio conditioning efforts using cardio exercise equipment largely depends on how dedicated, how hard, how long, and how often you exercise.

ABOUT THE AUTHOR

I didn't know much about exercise equipment until my uncle who is getting up in age needed to buy a cardio workout equipment and asked me to help him find one that would be good for him. That's where it all started. I did some research and my goodness! - There are so many things that should be taken into consideration that I had really never given thought to. The more I found out, the more I needed to find out.

I thought to myself if I found out all this stuff, surely other exercise equipment buyers would want to know this information too so that they can make an informed decision. So that was the birth of my book. I guess it was kind of a fun project to do. No deadlines or anything like that. I took my time and it's finally done now. Hopefully others will benefit from the research. My uncle has himself a real nice treadmill now as though it was just tailored for him. He's pretty happy about his purchase and I am too.